MERIDIAN MIDDLE SCHOOL
2195 Brandywyn Lane
Buffalo Grove, IL 60089

DISCARDED

LIVING WITH DISEASE

DIABETES

BY BILL McAULIFFE

CREATIVE 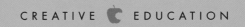 EDUCATION

Contents

In 1921, a young Canadian physician

named Frederick Banting created a summer job for himself: figuring out how to isolate and extract insulin, which was believed to control sugar levels in the blood, from the **pancreas** of a dog. The goal was to see whether the substance could stave off diabetes, then a fatal disease, in humans. Banting sought help from professor John Macleod at the University of Toronto, who provided him with an assistant, Charles Best, as well as a laboratory. By midsummer, Banting and Best's experiments of administering insulin were proving successful on diabetic dogs. In January 1922, the two researchers injected insulin into a Toronto boy who was dying of diabetes. Within two weeks, the boy was recovering. Later that year, Banting and Macleod published the first description of insulin's discovery, and the two shared the 1923 Nobel Prize in Physiology or Medicine for it. Their work remains one of the most dramatic medical breakthroughs of all time and continues to save millions of lives.

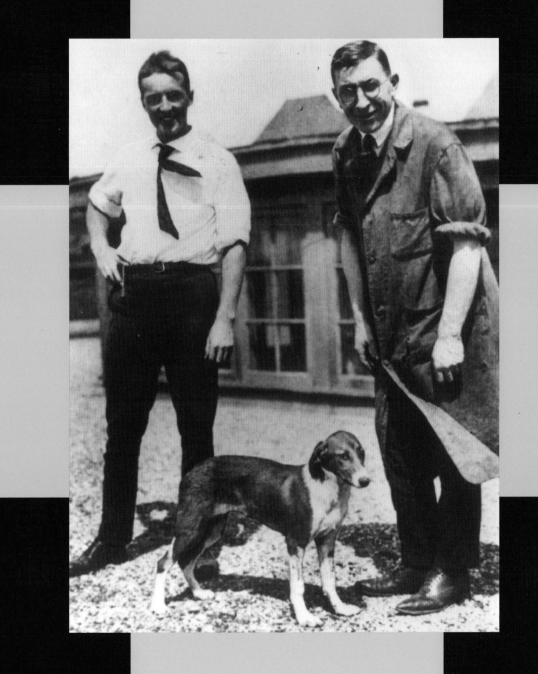

Charles Best (left) and Frederick Banting (right), pictured in 1921 with one of their canine patients.

CHAPTER ONE

THE SUGAR SICKNESS

Diabetes is an ancient enemy.

Egyptian and Greek physicians were acquainted with it thousands of years ago, recognizing the unquenchable thirst in its victims, as well as their continual need to urinate. In the second century A.D., the Greek physician Aretaeus of Cappadocia described the disease as "a melting down of the flesh and limbs into urine" and gave it the name diabetes, which is Greek for "a passer-through, or siphon," because of the near constant drawing off of urine from people who have the illness.

Convinced that urine might hold clues to understanding the condition, in the 1600s, London physician Thomas Willis actually tasted the urine of diabetes victims. Indeed, it began to reveal the story: the urine was sweet to the taste, suggesting that the disease was related to an excess of sugar. Later researchers would drip urine near an anthill; if ants were attracted to it, then the urine was sugary, and the person it came from probably had diabetes. The Latin word *mellitus*, meaning "honey sweet," was later attached to the disease's name. In time, it also became known as "the sugar sickness."

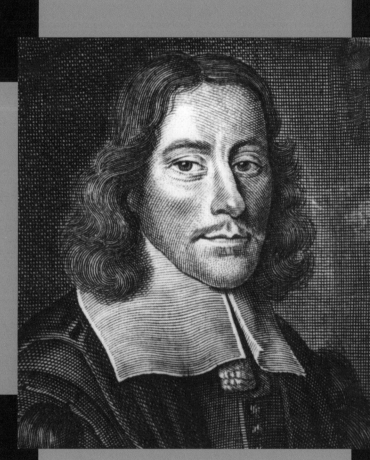

Thomas Willis was a physician to the English king, Charles I, in the 1640s and was later known for his research on the brain.

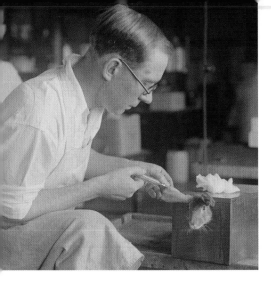

THE SUGAR SICKNESS

In the 1920s, insulin was extracted from certain animals and made into injectable doses for humans.

It wasn't until the late 1800s that European researchers determined that diabetes results from a body's failure to deliver sugar (glucose), derived from food, to cells, which need glucose's energy to function. In those days, having diabetes involved tremendous suffering. Patients often wasted away as their bodies were unable to convert food into nourishment the body could use. Despite this fact, during the early 1900s, some doctors tried to reduce the amount of glucose in diabetics' bloodstreams by prescribing a near-starvation diet. A key feature of the diet was a steep reduction in glucose-producing **carbohydrates**. This meant severely limiting the fruits, vegetables, and whole grains that diabetic patients could eat every day, as well as reducing the calories they got from other foods. When 14-year-old Elizabeth Hughes became one of the first patients to receive insulin for her diabetes in August 1922, her recovery included eating a piece of bread for the first time in 3 years.

Until that time, the life expectancy of someone diagnosed with diabetes was about one year. The restricted diet only prolonged a diabetic's decline. Patients' skin became hard and rough as damaged nerves stopped telling skin cells to produce the oils that keep the skin supple and healthy. In addition, acids built up in patients' blood, causing a distinctive, rotten-apple smell that often filled entire wards of hospitals where diabetics were treated. Patients in the advanced stages of diabetes, attempting to exhale the excess acids from their lungs, also tried to inhale more deeply, falling into a condition doctors called "air hunger" or "internal suffocation." If they'd lived long enough with the disease by then, they might also be suffering from blindness, heart problems, and infections. Ultimately, a patient would sink into a **coma** and die.

Great strides have been made in the past century in dealing with diabetes. The most important of these was the discovery of insulin—both its role in the body's regulation of blood sugar and how to manufacture it. However, even Banting, the physician who discovered how to isolate and extract insulin from animals, cautioned that the substance was not a cure. Since his time, diabetes has continued to spread rapidly around the world. According to the World Health Organization (WHO), about 30 million people worldwide had diabetes in 1985. A decade later, the number was estimated to be 135 million. The latest estimate of the number of people with diabetes worldwide is 285 million. Today, 23.6 million people in the United States and more than 3 million in Canada have diabetes. It is the seventh-leading cause of death in America, claiming 72,500 lives annually, and contributes to the deaths of more than 41,500

In the U.S., African Americans, American Indians, and Hispanics are at least twice as likely to have type 2 diabetes as non-Hispanic white people are. In fact, more than 15 percent of American Indians have diabetes, one of the highest rates of incidence out of any ethnic group in the world.

Canadians each year. By 2030, at least 435 million people around the world are expected to have diabetes. The Centers for Disease Control and Prevention predicts that, by 2050, as many as 1 in 3 American adults could have diabetes, up from 1 in 10 in 2010. Aging, unhealthy diets, obesity, and increasingly **sedentary** lifestyles will all contribute to more cases of diabetes.

Diabetes isn't contagious. But some ethnic and racial groups are more vulnerable to it than others. African Americans, Hispanics, and American Indians have much higher rates of diabetes than do whites. Family history can also make some people more vulnerable. But a far more significant risk factor is excess weight. Most people who are diagnosed with type 2 diabetes (as opposed to type 1) are overweight or **obese**. That suggests that the lifestyles of people in countries with rich diets and a relative lack of exercise are key contributors to diabetes.

Because it's a chronic (long-lasting) disease without a cure, a diagnosis of diabetes can be difficult for some people to hear, since it means adopting new routines that they'll have to follow for the rest of their lives. National Football League quarterback Jay Cutler said being diagnosed with diabetes after his third season of professional football was "overwhelming." Cutler had lost 35 pounds (16 kg) during the

Starring with Diabetes

In 1969, Mary Tyler Moore was a 32-year-old, Emmy-award-winning television star about to launch her own show. Then, after miscarrying a pregnancy, a blood test determined she had type 1 diabetes. In the years since, she has developed a range of diabetes-related complications, including nerve damage in her feet and deterioration in her eyes, to the point where she needs help walking through dimly lit backstage clutter. But she has continued to act on stage and in films, winning several Tony Awards for her performances on Broadway and being nominated for an Oscar. Since 1984 she has been chairperson of the Juvenile Diabetes Research Foundation. "Spontaneity is one of the first of life's pleasures that's lost when diabetes appears," she writes in her book *Growing Up Again*. But regulation is a skill all diabetics must learn to survive, she adds. "If you don't control diabetes, it will control you."

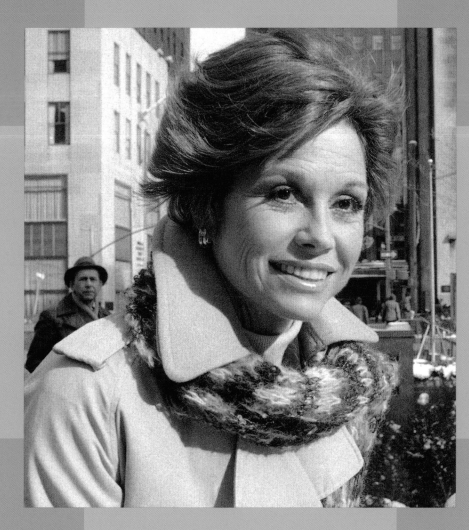

Mary Tyler Moore,
pictured about 10
years after her
diabetes diagnosis.

2007 season while playing for the Denver Broncos. A blood test some months later confirmed that he had diabetes. With insulin doses and a more regulated diet, Cutler regained half of his lost weight in the month after his diagnosis. By 2009, he was serving as the starting quarterback for the Chicago Bears. "It's a big adjustment," Cutler said shortly after finding out he had diabetes. "You're 25 years old, you're used to eating whatever you want, doing whatever you want…. But it's something you have to deal with. This is a serious, serious disease, and I'm going to have it for the rest of my life."

Cutler joined a list of well-known athletes who have reached the top levels of their sports despite having diabetes: baseball's Jackie Robinson, tennis's Billie Jean King, boxing's Joe Frazier, and hockey's Bobby Clarke, among others. U.S. Supreme Court Justice Sonia Sotomayor has had diabetes since she was eight years old. Actress Halle Berry is another diabetic. Notable American diabetics of the past include Nobel Prize–winning novelist Ernest Hemingway, singer Elvis Presley, author Laura Ingalls Wilder, and inventor Thomas Edison.

Opposite page, clockwise from left: Jackie Robinson, Elvis Presley, Halle Berry, and Jay Cutler.

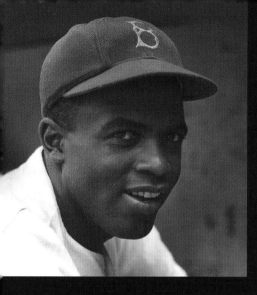

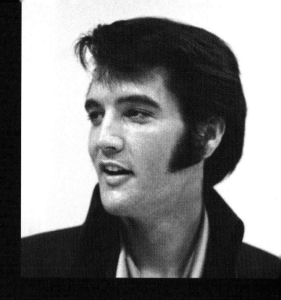

About 0.2 percent of people under the age of 20 in the U.S. have diabetes. The figure jumps to 2.6 percent for people between 20 and 39 years of age. Of those 40 to 59 years old, 10.8 percent have the disease, while 23 percent of those 60 and older have diabetes.

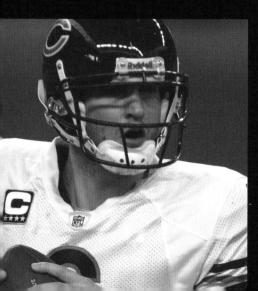

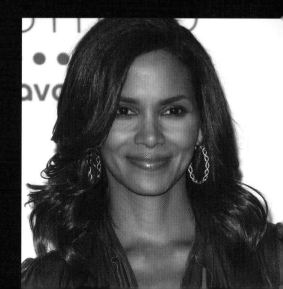

CHAPTER TWO

TYPES AND CAUSES

Diabetes puts a person's body at war with itself. Normally, when a person digests food, the liver distributes glucose from the food into the blood. Glucose is a basic fuel for the body, but it needs some help to get into cells. In a healthy person, the **hormone** insulin, produced in the pancreas, opens up receptors on the cells that allow glucose to enter.

In a person with diabetes, the body fails to move the glucose from the blood into the cells, either because the pancreas stops producing insulin or because the cells become **resistant** to insulin's effects and don't allow the glucose to enter. As a result, glucose builds up in the blood. The kidneys try to dilute the glucose by drawing water out of cells. This causes the diabetic to urinate frequently and to become tremendously thirsty because he's becoming dehydrated. He also develops an intense hunger because his cells aren't getting any glucose from the foods he has eaten. These are the key outward symptoms of diabetes.

A person whose pancreas generates too little insulin or none at all suffers from type 1 diabetes, which is also known as "insulin-dependent"

In a healthy kidney, blood that is carried through it is filtered by clusters of capillaries called glomeruli.

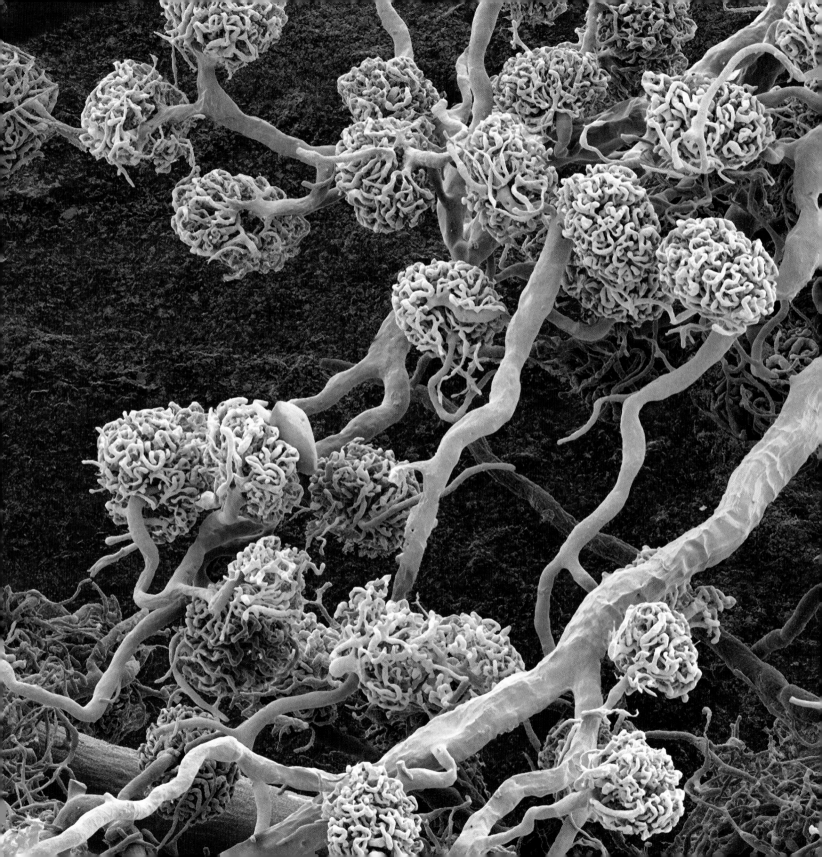

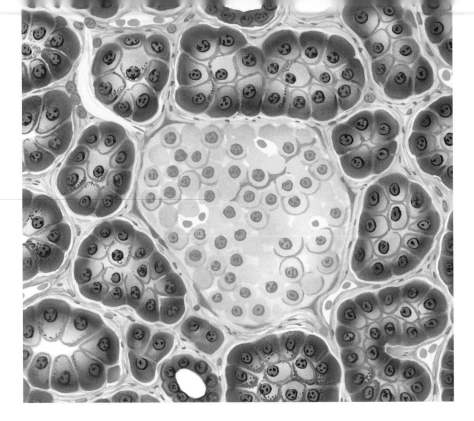

Regular pancreas cells surround the insulin-producing cells called the islets of Langerhans.

diabetes, since its victims must take insulin by injection or a pump. Type 1 diabetes most often appears in children and young adults, and its onset is usually sudden. It can be an **autoimmune** condition that develops following an illness such as pancreatitis, an inflammation of the pancreas that results when the body attacks a virus—normally a healthy response that in this case goes awry. Disorders of the **adrenal glands** and the **pituitary gland** and even medications a person takes for other diseases can cause type 1 diabetes, as can removal of the pancreas, which often results from cancer in that organ. Type 1 was previously known as juvenile diabetes, but its onset can occur at any age, and those who have the disease as children often carry it into adulthood.

A person whose blood cells are resistant to insulin and thus can't absorb glucose has type 2 diabetes. Type 2 was formerly known as "adult-onset" diabetes, since it was most commonly diagnosed in adults. But children are increasingly being diagnosed with this form of the disease as well. It's not clear why some people's cells become resistant to insulin. Some suspected causes include an unhealthy lifestyle, an infection or illness that damages the pancreas, changes in the levels of other hormones in the body, and alcohol abuse.

Although type 2 diabetes is more likely to be **hereditary** than type 1, it is more often linked to behavioral factors, particularly poor diet, lack of exercise, and excess weight. More than 90 percent of the people with diabetes in the U.S. have type 2. People with type 2 diabetes can often control their symptoms by eating more healthful food, exercising more, and losing weight. They usually don't require regular doses of insulin, as people with type 1 do.

Latent autoimmune diabetes in adults (LADA) can be misdiagnosed as being type 2, since it is often caught in patients 25 years of age or older. Also like type 2, LADA can be controlled with diet at the onset, but over time, the patient becomes dependent on insulin. This causes LADA to be categorized as a form of type 1 diabetes.

A Brother's Song

At the age of 13, Nick Jonas, a singer, guitarist, and drummer with the Jonas Brothers, had fame and wealth most teenagers could only dream of. He also had diabetes. Before being diagnosed with type 1 diabetes in 2005, Jonas had never had any serious health problems, and the news was such a shock that he wondered if he could continue with his music career. But before long he was back on tour, managing his blood sugar with an insulin pump. In 2007, Jonas announced publicly that he was a diabetic, and since then, he has used his celebrity status to focus attention on diabetes research and care. Jonas emphasized that young people with the disease needed to find ways to stay positive, avoid depression, and find support from family and friends. His song "A Little Bit Longer" was about being diagnosed and living with the disease.

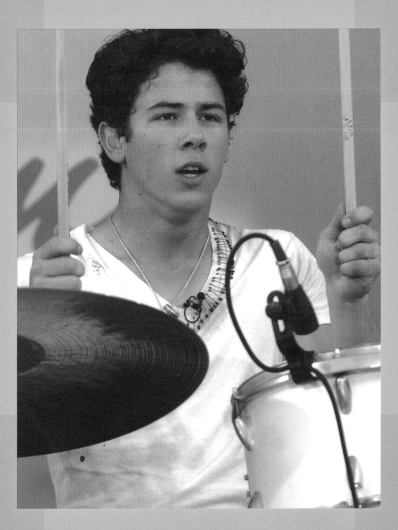

In 2010, Nick Jonas toured with his brothers, Joe and Kevin, and singer Demi Lovato.

Another fairly common type of diabetes, gestational diabetes, affects pregnant women. Hormones that are important for a baby's growth also sometimes limit the effects of insulin in transporting glucose to the mother's cells, which is how she can develop diabetes. Gestational diabetes vanishes when the baby is born, but a mother then has a 40 to 60 percent risk of developing type 2 diabetes within 5 to 10 years, compared with a 15 percent risk for the general population. However, the risk that the baby will develop the disease solely due to the mother's gestational diabetes is small.

Pre-diabetes is a condition related to diabetes, but it is not as dangerous. Pre-diabetes, which afflicts an estimated 57 million American adults, is characterized by higher-than-normal blood glucose levels that are not quite high enough to lead to a diagnosis of diabetes. Despite its name, pre-diabetes may not ever result in diabetes, and it doesn't require the same level of aggressive response. Still, if a pre-diabetic doesn't take the steps to prevent it, pre-diabetes may progress to type 2 diabetes within 10 years. But whether they develop diabetes or not, people with pre-diabetes face some of the same complications as do patients with diabetes, such as an increased risk of stroke and heart disease.

If diabetes isn't controlled, it can create several often disabling conditions in people. When a person's body can't use glucose for energy

A child of a type 2 diabetic parent has an 8 to 15 percent chance of getting the disease. If both parents or a brother or sister have it, the risk can approach 50 percent. An identical twin with diabetes boosts the risk toward 75 or even 90 percent, but that chance declines with age.

About 6.4 percent of adults worldwide have diabetes, according to the International Diabetes Federation. Regional diabetes rates range from 5 percent in the Western Pacific—which includes China, Japan, and the Pacific Islands—to 11.7 in North America and 3.2 in Africa. The global rate is expected to be 7.8 percent by 2030.

because there is too much sugar in the bloodstream (which is then diluted and expelled as urine), it tries to make up for it by converting fats and **proteins** into energy instead. This process causes acid compounds called ketones to form fatty byproducts in the blood, leading to a condition called ketoacidosis. Symptoms of ketoacidosis include fruity-smelling breath, trouble breathing, difficulty concentrating, or vomiting. A person with ketoacidosis needs to drink plenty of water and get medical help immediately, because the condition can lead to a coma and even death.

Too little glucose in the blood causes a condition called hypoglycemia. Skipping or delaying meals, eating too few carbohydrates, or exercising too long or strenuously can cause this condition. It can also result from taking too much insulin. Early signs of hypoglycemia include cold sweats, weakness, shakiness, dizziness, and headache. It can also cause slurred speech and behavior that resembles drunkenness. Left untreated, hypoglycemia can lead to a dangerous condition known as insulin shock, which is caused by an imbalance between the amounts of insulin and glucose in the blood. Insulin shock can result in seizures, comas, or even death. But hypoglycemia can be kept from progressing to insulin shock by drinking sugary soda or fruit juice or eating hard candy—part of the survival kit many diabetics carry with them every day.

CHAPTER THREE

MANAGING LIFE

Although diabetes was once a common

killer, today it is managed successfully through continual blood testing, medication, diet, and exercise. But diabetics must be disciplined about controlling their condition. Without constant monitoring, diabetes can lead to an array of serious health complications and even death.

Some types of nerve endings in the skin, such as those in fingertips (pictured opposite), are responsible for the sensation of touch.

Excessive glucose in the blood can draw fluid out of the lenses in the eye, causing blurred vision. Other eye problems such as **cataracts** and **glaucoma** can result from diabetes. A more serious complication is diabetic **retinopathy**, in which blood vessels enlarge or become blocked and leak fluid into the retina. In extreme cases, diabetes can even cause blindness.

Diabetes also frequently leads to a condition called **peripheral** neuropathy, in which nerve endings, especially those in the legs and feet, lose their sensitivity. As a result, a diabetic may not feel a blister, cut, or other minor foot injury, which might cause it to become infected. This can lead to rotting tissue and the need to amputate toes, feet, or legs.

Diabetes is also a leading cause of kidney disease and often causes obstructions in **arteries**, increasing the risk of heart attack and stroke.

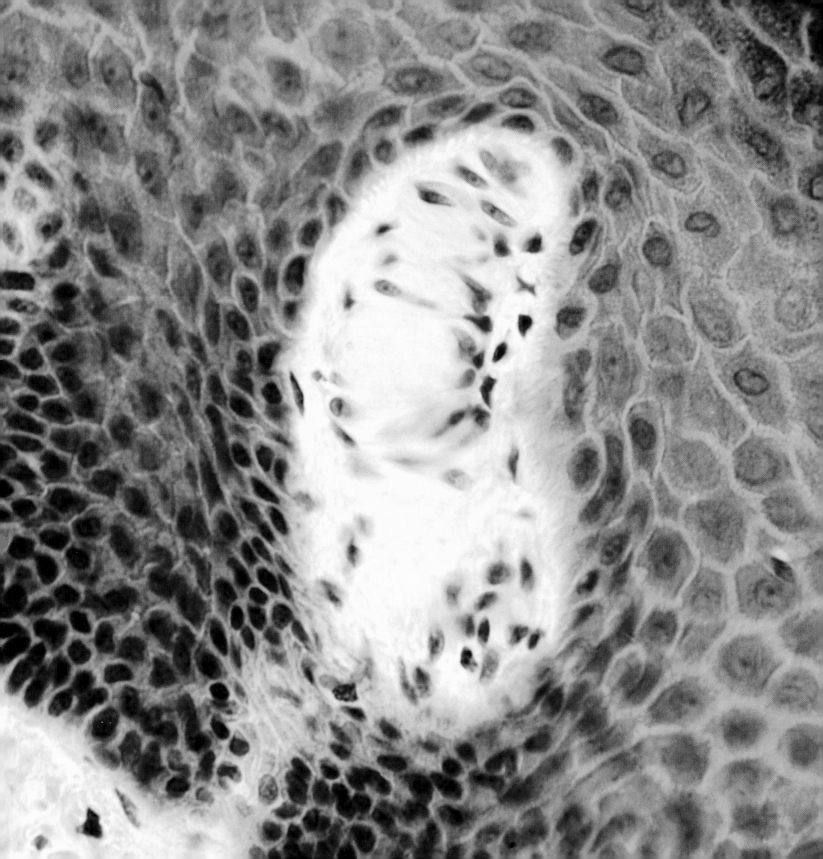

An Island of Diabetics

Nauru, in the Pacific Ocean, is the world's smallest island nation. But it has one of the world's biggest diabetes problems. For centuries, residents of the eight-square-mile (21 sq km) island lived simply, enjoying a diet of fresh-caught fish and homegrown fruit and vegetables. That isolated and uncomplicated lifestyle changed forever in the early 1900s. The discovery and subsequent mining of phosphate, a mineral valued as a fertilizer, transformed Nauru briefly into one of the world's richest nations. However, it also wiped out most of its cropland, requiring the people to begin importing most of their food. The imported food contained far more sweeteners and fats than Nauruans were used to. Today, about 31 percent of the nation's nearly 9,000 adults have diabetes, and about 80 percent of Nauruans are obese, one of the highest rates for a particular group of people in the world.

Mining for phosphate on Nauru involves digging around ancient coral reefs that are found underground.

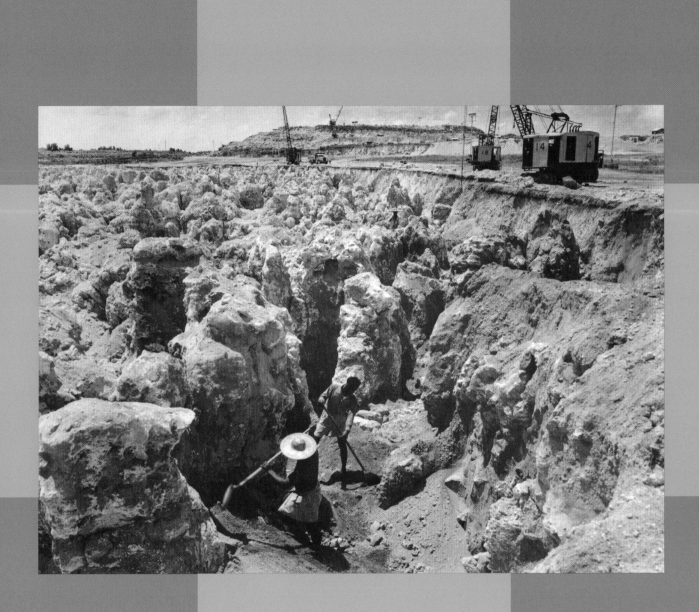

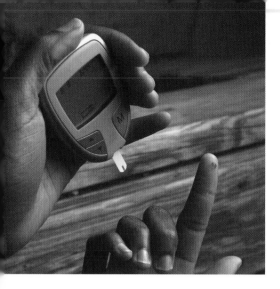

It takes only one drop of blood to test glucose concentration on a handheld monitor.

Researchers are also investigating possible links between diabetes and **Alzheimer's disease**.

To prevent the disease from causing such complications, diabetics have to test their blood glucose level frequently. Many diabetics check their blood glucose level shortly after each meal; some, if they're prone to hypoglycemia, check it each time they get into a car to drive or operate other such machinery. Blood glucose is usually measured in milligrams per deciliter (mg/dl). In a healthy person, the blood glucose concentration is usually 70 to 130 mg/dl before meals and less than 140 mg/dl 2 hours after meals. Readings above 200 on repeated tests are often the first definite indication of diabetes. But some people have readings of 600 or 700 when diabetes is first diagnosed.

To check their blood glucose level, diabetics usually use a small blade, sometimes spring-loaded, to quickly draw a drop of blood, most often from a fingertip. The blood gets applied to a paper strip, which is then inserted into a blood glucose monitor, a battery-operated device about the size of a cell phone. The monitor displays the level of glucose concentration in the blood. Diabetics can also monitor their blood glucose continuously with electronic devices worn on their bodies. One, worn like a wristwatch, sends electric currents through the skin to detect glucose levels. Another uses a needlelike sensor inserted under the skin. Most of these monitors can also sound alarms when glucose gets too high or too low. In addition to testing their blood themselves, diabetics also take a glucose test, called the A1C, at a laboratory several times a year to determine their average blood glucose level over the span of the previous three months.

But knowing how much glucose is in their blood is only the beginning for diabetics. Patients must then adjust their glucose level to keep it in the range their doctor recommends. Type 1 diabetics do this by taking insulin. In most cases, a diabetic injects insulin several times a day—depending on her blood glucose level—with a syringe and needle. The best place for injections is an area of loose skin, usually the abdomen. Some insulin dosages take effect within 5 minutes and last 3 to 4 hours; others take 6 hours or more to begin working but remain effective for 24 hours. Diabetics can also take insulin with a pen-like device that forces insulin through the skin without use of a needle or even an inhaler. Increasingly, a diabetic's preferred device is a pocket-sized pump, strapped to an arm or leg or even attached to a belt loop at the waist, that administers insulin throughout the day through a needle inserted under the skin. Pumps are often ideal for teenagers because they can respond to teens' irregular schedules and can be concealed, eliminating possible embarrassment.

Type 2 diabetics often control their blood sugar by designing and following a specific diet. Diabetics try to eat meals at the same times each day to help regulate blood glucose levels. That's why traveling or dining out can be troublesome for diabetics. But the most complicated challenge diabetes presents may be to families of diabetic kids who, like all kids, want to snack, try different foods, eat a lot (or nothing at all), and eat with their friends. "Arguments about food can disrupt the daily life and harmony of the family," writes dietician and diabetes educator Betty Page Brackenridge. "Families go to war over how many vanilla wafers were eaten after school."

Meals for diabetics don't have to be boring—just healthful. They generally consist of what anyone would recognize as a "balanced" diet, with small portions that might also help a person lose weight. An ideal dinner plate for a diabetic would be filled half with vegetables, one-fourth with meat or fish, and one-fourth with whole grains or beans, peas, or lentils. Sweets are allowed, but they might have to take the place of some

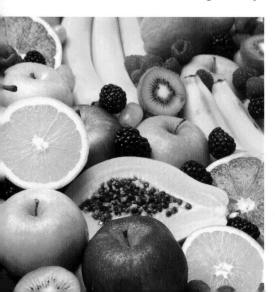

Fresh fruit is a healthy substitute for processed foods that may contain too much sugar for a diabetic to eat.

The Body Mass Index (BMI) combines height with weight to determine whether a person's body is normal, overweight, obese, or extremely obese. BMI is determined by dividing one's weight in kilograms (pounds x 0.45) by one's height in meters squared. A BMI greater than 30 is generally considered obese.

Diabetes is linked to many other serious health problems. More than 60 percent of leg and foot amputations that aren't the result of accident or injury are performed on diabetics. Diabetics have two to four times the heart disease death rates and two to four times the stroke risk of adults without diabetes.

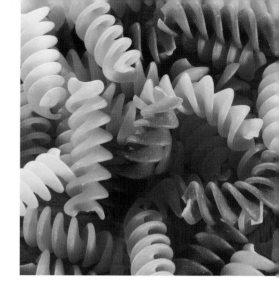

carbohydrates—two cookies instead of a piece of bread, for example—since both produce blood glucose. The ideal diet for a diabetic depends on what type of diabetes she has, as well as on her body size, muscle mass, and other factors, including her activity level. A type 1 diabetic who is not trying to lose weight is advised to keep her total caloric intake to 16 calories per pound (0.45 kg) of body weight. For a 150-pound (68 kg) person, that would be 2,400 calories a day. People with type 2 diabetes are advised to hold that to 1,500 to 1,800 calories per day. About half the calories should come from carbohydrates.

Diabetics must quickly learn how to read food and nutrition labels and to find where sugar can hide in otherwise healthy foods. They have to use their math skills almost constantly throughout the day, calculating their intake of sugar, carbohydrates, calories, and fats. Creative food-swapping often helps a diabetic make the numbers balance. Living with diabetes may often seem like an endless process of calculations, combined with a level of self-discipline few non-diabetics can understand, but it all adds up to a healthier life.

Pasta contains complex carbohydrates, which release energy slowly instead of providing a quick burst of sugar.

CHAPTER FOUR

STILL SEEKING A CURE

Few scientific discoveries have been

as dramatic as the isolation of insulin at the University of Toronto in 1921. It allowed people who were near death from diabetes, even in a coma, to recover. Insulin is necessary to fight diabetes, but it is not a cure. Researchers continue to develop other medications and technologies that could significantly improve the lives of people with diabetes.

At an English hospital in the 1940s, children were taught how to administer their own insulin.

While researchers knew almost a century ago that insulin could help reverse the ravages of diabetes, they didn't know why. It wasn't until the late 1940s that scientists discovered that insulin acts like a key to allow glucose into cells. A few years later, a French **pharmacologist** named Marcel Janbon was researching a group of drugs that had been used to fight bacterial infections and accidentally found that they could help a person's pancreas manufacture more insulin. These drugs, called sulfonyl-ureas, helped reduce the amount of insulin many diabetics had to take by injection and were the first oral drug, or pill, used to control diabetes.

At that time, patients used insulin from cows and pigs, which, while similar to human insulin, sometimes provoked an allergic reaction.

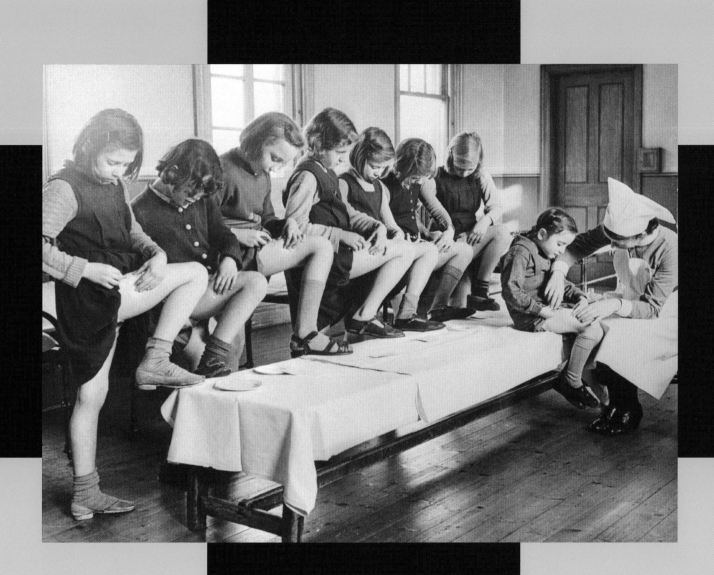

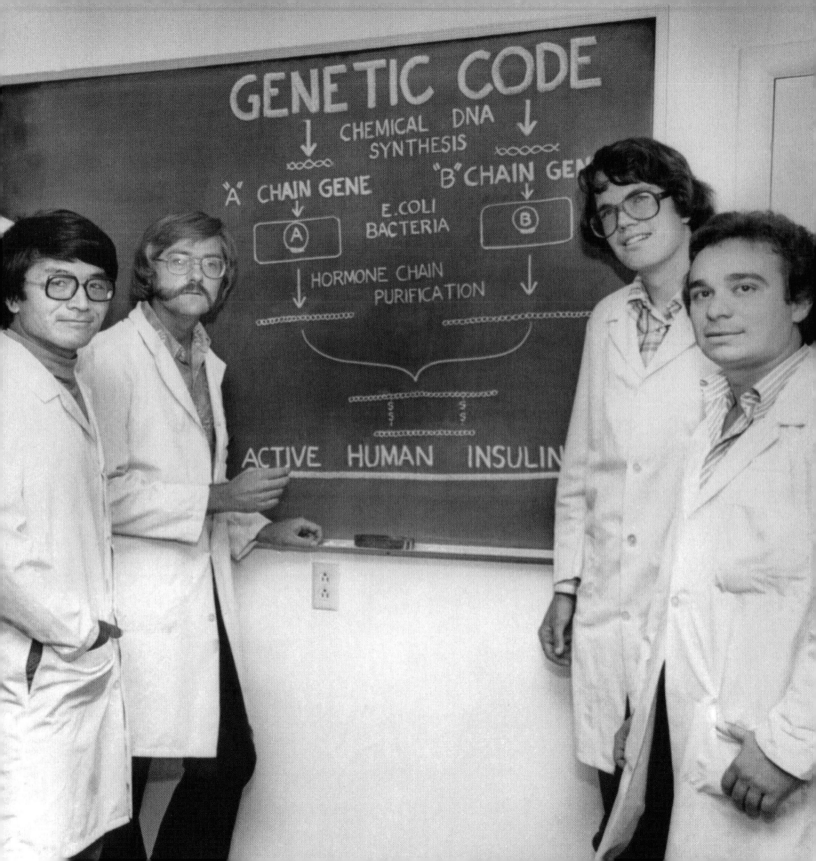

It took nearly 30 more years before researchers discovered that when the human **gene** that produces insulin was inserted into cells of E. coli bacteria, the bacteria produced insulin in great quantities. The purified manufactured insulin was cheaper to produce than animal insulin, and today it is the most commonly used form of the hormone.

In 1994, another medication, called metformin, was approved for use in the U.S. When a person is at rest, or not eating, the liver continues to release glucose into the bloodstream. That's one likely reason why diabetics often find their blood sugar levels high in the morning, a situation called the "dawn effect." Metformin slows this release and has the added benefits of reducing fat levels in the blood and promoting weight loss. In a research study published in 2002, participants with pre-diabetes who took metformin reduced their risk of progressing to type 2 diabetes by 31 percent, compared with those who took no medications or other action.

Several other oral medications with clear benefits for patients with type 2 diabetes have been approved within the last 15 years. One group of oral medications lowers insulin resistance in cells, which could allow type 2 diabetics who are on insulin to reduce their need for the hormone, while also increasing levels of a beneficial type of **cholesterol** in the

Scientists demonstrate how their combined efforts in genetic engineering resulted in the first artificially produced human insulin.

blood. Another group of drugs blocks some starch-digestion after meals, limiting the usual increase in blood sugar and thus the need for insulin or the risk of hyperglycemia (too much sugar). However, many of these drugs have unhealthy side effects, including stomach irritation and weight gain—often the opposite of what a diabetic is trying to achieve.

Not all diabetes research focuses on medication. Diet and exercise have long been seen as critical factors in blunting the effects of diabetes. From 2001 to 2002, separate studies conducted in the U.S. and Finland showed that people with pre-diabetes who cut down on the fat and calories in their diets and exercised two and a half hours per week reduced their risk of developing diabetes by 58 percent. In the U.S. study, participants who were 60 and older saw even greater benefits, with a reduced risk of 71 percent. While weight loss through exercise is beneficial to almost all overweight people because it helps the body work more efficiently, diabetes researchers believe that for people with type 2 diabetes, exercise itself helps make one's cells more receptive to insulin, enabling them to absorb energy-producing glucose from the blood.

In patients with type 1 diabetes that has advanced to the point of causing other serious disabilities such as eye, skin, circulatory, and nerve damage, or kidney failure, a pancreas transplant represents a

Medical treatment for those diagnosed with diabetes cost $174 billion in the U.S. in 2007, up 33 percent from 2002. Of that, $58 billion was for lost work time, disability, or premature death. On average, a diabetic's annual medical costs are 2.3 times higher than those of a person without diabetes.

After 20 years with type 1 diabetes, nearly all people with the disease develop some form of retinopathy, compromising their vision, and more than half of those with type 2 diabetes follow the same course. Diabetic retinopathy is the most frequent cause of new blindness among adults ages 20 to 74.

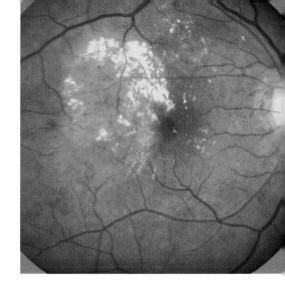

cure. But this type of transplantation requires major surgery and is usually performed at the same time as or just after a kidney transplant. The patient's existing pancreas is often left in place because it may still be making digestive juices and be able to aid in digestion. In a kidney-pancreas transplant, there is double the normal risk that the patient's immune system will reject the foreign organs. However, in 72 percent of patients who undergo a double transplant, the new pancreas continues to function for 5 years; about 52 percent of those who receive only a pancreas see the same results. An alternative strategy is the transplantation of islet cells, which produce insulin in the pancreas. But this, too, is complicated surgery, requiring strong drugs to keep the body's immune system from rejecting the new materials. There is also a relatively small supply of donors.

Researchers are continuing to look into whether a **vaccine** might be developed to help children who may be genetically prone to diabetes avoid the disease. Meanwhile, insulin obtained from genetically modified plants such as safflower, lettuce, and even tobacco is currently being tested in humans. It could make insulin more available to meet what is expected to be a growing demand worldwide.

An image of the eye showing the leakage of fluid and collection of protein deposits that indicate retinopathy.

At the same time, researchers are trying to develop what could be a breakthrough piece of technology: an artificial pancreas. Such a device, which would secrete insulin into the bloodstream, would dramatically ease the burden of blood testing and insulin injections and remove the risk of mistakes. Researchers believe the artificial pancreas will be available to the public as a treatment option by 2015.

Even as researchers continue to look for ways to treat diabetes, they're also probing into questions far beyond the disease itself, studying depression and other complications, possible connections between diabetes and other diseases, and environmental risk factors such as exposure to viruses and even to cold weather.

Yet scientists remain largely baffled as to the disease's cause. In 2008, researchers identified 6 new genes (adding to the 10 previously found) that might have a role in causing diabetes, but no one knows for certain why some people get it and others—even those with common risk factors—do not. What is encouraging, however, is that while diabetes is on the rise, it is also becoming more manageable. With new drugs and technology, combined with better nutrition, diabetics are living longer, more balanced, and less disrupted lives than ever before.

First in Care

Elliott P. Joslin was studying at Yale University in the late 1880s when his aunt was diagnosed with diabetes. He began to research the little-known but devastating disease at Harvard Medical School several years later and kept patient records so extensive that insurance companies later used them to file claims. Joslin's exhaustive work with patients helped establish the foundation of standard diabetes treatment, emphasizing a restricted diet and exercise. (He later added insulin to that strategy.) Joslin was able to show that adjustments in diet and exercise reduced diabetes death rates by 20 percent. In 1916, he published the first manual outlining how patients could manage their own diabetes. The manual is still in print. Joslin founded the world's first clinic for diabetes care in Boston in 1898. Despite his efforts to curtail the disease, nearly 50 years later Joslin was one of the first researchers to identify diabetes as an **epidemic** in the U.S.

GLOSSARY

adrenal glands: glands located on top of the kidneys that produce body chemicals that respond to stress

Alzheimer's disease: a condition, most often found in older people, in which brain matter and mental function are destroyed

arteries: blood vessels, or tubes, that carry blood away from the heart to other parts of the body

autoimmune: relating to a response in which the body attacks parts of itself to protect against a larger threat, such as a virus or disease

carbohydrates: foods, such as potatoes, pasta, and beans, in which carbon, hydrogen, and oxygen combine to make sugars, starches, and other substances

cataracts: cloudy areas on the lenses of the eyes that limit sight

cholesterol: a soft, waxy substance found in the bloodstream and all cells that is used to help digest fats and strengthen cell membranes; it can cause heart problems when it builds up in the blood

coma: a state of deep unconsciousness caused by disease, injury, or poison, in which a person is unable to see or hear what is going on around him or her

epidemic: a disease that has spread rapidly through a segment of the population in a given geographic area

gene: the basic unit of instruction in a cell, which controls a person's physical traits and passes characteristics from parents to offspring

glaucoma: a condition characterized by high blood pressure within the eye, which can damage vision

hereditary: passed on from parents to children through the genes

hormone: a substance produced by the body that affects activity within the body, such as growth

latent: existing in a hidden or inactive form

obese: having a body mass index greater than 30, which is a measurement of one's weight in relation to height

pancreas: a large gland near the intestines that aids in digestion and produces insulin

peripheral: distant from the center or core

pharmacologist: a person who studies drugs and their therapeutic use

pituitary gland: a gland at the base of the brain that produces chemicals to help control basic body functions such as growth, blood pressure, and conversion of food into energy, as well as the growth and development of other glands

proteins: complex structures that are the basic components of all living cells

resistant: unaffected by the harmful effects of something, such as a drug

retinopathy: a degenerative disease of the retina, the light-sensitive part of the eye that receives an image and sends it to the brain

sedentary: characterized by a lack of physical activity

vaccine: a substance given in a shot or by mouth that helps the immune system form antibodies (disease-fighting proteins) to fight off a specific disease

BIBLIOGRAPHY

American Diabetes Association. "Diabetes Basics." American Diabetes Association. http://www.diabetes.org/diabetes-basics.

———. *American Diabetes Association Complete Guide to Diabetes.* Alexandria, Va.: American Diabetes Association, 2005.

Bliss, Michael. *The Discovery of Insulin.* Chicago: University of Chicago Press, 2007.

Colberg, Sheri. *Diabetic Athlete's Handbook.* Champaign, Ill.: Human Kinetics, 2009.

Collazo-Clavell, Maria, ed. *Mayo Clinic: The Essential Diabetes Book.* New York: Time, 2009.

Longe, Jacqueline, ed. *The Gale Encyclopedia of Medicine.* Detroit: Thomson Gale, 2006.

Moore, Mary Tyler. *Growing Up Again: Confronting My Diabetes.* New York: St. Martin's Press, 2009.

National Diabetes Information Clearinghouse. "Diabetes Overview." National Institute of Diabetes and Digestive and Kidney Diseases. http://diabetes.niddk.nih.gov/dm/pubs/overview.

FURTHER READING

Haney, Johannah. *Juvenile Diabetes.* New York: Benchmark Books, 2005.

Hyde, Margaret, and Elizabeth Forsyth. *Diabetes.* New York: Franklin Watts, 2003.

Loughrey, Anita. *Explaining Diabetes.* North Mankato, Minn.: Smart Apple Media, 2010.

Stoyles, Pennie. *The A–Z of Health.* Vol. 2, *C–E.* North Mankato, Minn.: Smart Apple Media, 2011.

INDEX

Published by Creative Education • P.O. Box 227, Mankato, Minnesota 56002
Creative Education is an imprint of The Creative Company
www.thecreativecompany.us
Design and production by The Design Lab • Art direction by Rita Marshall
Printed by Corporate Graphics in the United States of America
Photographs by Alamy (Medicalpicture, Phototake Inc.), AP Images (Marty Lederhandler), Corbis (Bettmann, Visuals Unlimited), Getty Images (Mark Davis, Steve Gschmeissner/SPL, Hulton Archive, Kevin Mazur/WireImage, Michael Ochs Archives, Gregory Shamus), iStockphoto (Mark Hatfield, Morgan Lane Studios, StockStudios)

Library of Congress Cataloging-in-Publication Data
McAuliffe, Bill. Diabetes / by Bill McAuliffe. p. cm. — (Living with disease)
Includes bibliographical references and index. Summary: A look at diabetes, examining the ways in which the disease develops, its different forms and symptoms, the effects it has on a person's daily life, and improvements in methods of treatment.
ISBN 978-1-60818-074-5
1. Diabetes—Juvenile literature. I. Title. II. Series.
RC660.5.M33 2011   616.4'62—dc22   2010030364

CPSIA: 110310 PO1384
First Edition 9 8 7 6 5 4 3 2 1